"WEIGHT LOSS, SHEDDING OFF THE POUNDS",

TABLE OF CONTENTS

INTRODUCTION

From the 1970s to date, more and more people have continued to fall victim of the "obese" tag. Weight loss has risen in stature to become the most talked about health issue in the last half a century. Books have been written, courses produced and videos made to provide an answer to the yearning of individuals looking to shed off a few extra pounds here and there.

Within this time, weight loss has grown into a multibillion-dollar industry. Yet, in spite of significant research and scientific studies by the day, more people continue to fail at the weight loss game. The reasons are not far-fetched. Aside from the fact that weight loss requires the right motivation, there is as much confusion as there is actual, workable knowledge.

There are just too many magic-fix solutions out there. Sadly, most of these solutions prove to be useless and even harmful to users some of the time. Instead of turning inwards to look at our lifestyle, most of them try to reverse-engineer biochemical processes in the body or interfere with some of our nutrition cycles to force weight loss. However, weight loss cannot and should not be forced. Forcing yourself physically through starvation or biochemically is bound to backfire and cause relapses. Instead, the secret to weight loss has been handed down to us by our ancestors, the earliest men.

Two, three hundred years ago, obesity was not the problem it used to be. In truth, it was even considered a sign of affluence in some societies. More importantly though, it was less rampant than now. Go back a millennium, and you will find out that there is hardly any mention of obesity at all. How then did obesity come to be such a common fixture of life today?

The secret is in our lifestyle choices regarding food and physical activity. Early man fed on a natural diet that provided him with only the most needed nutrients for his sustenance. Food for the early man was a question of survival and not the indulgence we have turned it to today. It wasn't a panacea to his sweet tooth problem; food to him was just as essential as sleep. So, he ate but only in such quantities and varieties as his body needed. No more, no less. By eating naturally and selectively, our ancestors made sure they didn't consume extraneous substances and nutrients that could affect normal metabolism in their bodies.

That was not all. As hunters and gatherers, each day was filled with enough activities to burn off whatever food they didn't need within their body systems. There was never any chance of excess food getting stored as fat deposits because their daily rate of activity didn't leave that chance. Three centuries ago, people certainly engaged in more physical activity. There was hardly any profession that required you to sit in one place for long. Even if it did, people got to other places by walking or riding horses, good, old physical activities on their own.

Today, the rise of technology has changed things. We live in so much technology-sponsored comfort that we no longer get the kind of exercise our ancestors got from their daily activities. Now, we drive, fly and get ferried around by different applications of technology. It is something to be grateful for, but when you ally our weird nutritional choices with a chronic shortage of physical activity, you begin to get a picture that explains why obesity has become endemic.

That is what most quick-fix diets and weight loss programs don't tell you. To shed weight, beyond complicated diet plans, it is your nutrition and exercise that you must watch. I have written this book as a source of knowledge different from books in the same niche. The idea is not to give you a particular diet or tell you what nutrition plan to adopt. Instead, it is a book of knowledge concerning weight loss. You can then use this knowledge to select what diet plan would be most comfortable and efficient for your goals.

However, like Pablo Picasso, Italian master artist said, "Action is the foundational element of success" in whatever we aspire to do. Do not just read the tips within this book, put them to work to finally see some progress in your weight loss goal. Good luck!

CHAPTER ONE

DEMYSTIFYING OBESITY

The facts tell a grim story. Approximately 36% of Americans are grossly overweight. Worldwide, 39% of the world's population above eighteen years old, representing close to two billion people, are grossly overweight; of this number, 13% are already obese. Coupled with the attendant dangers of lugging around extra pounds that are not needed, obesity has rightly occupied a frontline place in health discussions globally. But what is obesity?

Forgive me if I do not give you a textbook dictionary; you can get that from a dictionary. Instead, technically, a person is deemed obese if they have a body mass index (BMI) greater than 30. What is BMI? A person's BMI is determined by dividing his/her weight in kilogram by the square of his height in meters.

A BMI below 25 is considered best and healthiest for metabolism. A BMI value above 25 is qualified as overweight, and anything above 30 requires the tag obesity, as I mentioned earlier. This book promised to talk about obesity, but the simple truth is that there is very little difference between being overweight and obese. Both states require immediate work to lose weight and gain a better life.

Between 1975 and 2016, research indicated that the number of obese people worldwide tripled in adults. Even more alarmingly, the prevalence in children more than quadrupled from 4% to about 18%. Yet, within this same period, funding and research on obesity have increased significantly. What does this tell us?

It means that we are either not getting the required empirical data we need or the vast majority of people are not doing what they should be doing. The latter is the actual truth. Yes, there are various conflicting reports out there, but we already have the knowledge that matters; eat right, exercise adequately. That is simply the secret to weight loss.

However, eating right is not the easiest decision to come to after the vast majority of people have been raised on a pretty careless diet that cared less for health and placed more on culinary accomplishments. Society has taught most of us to look out for the quality in taste, and fulfil our common desires, rather than the health value of what we are eating. Therefore, when we feel like eating chocolate, we walk up to the mall and buy a large packet. When you go for lunch, you take wine in as much quantity as you feel like. When we feel thirsty, we pop a soda can instead of water.

The more we do this, the higher the chances that one begins to gather excess fat. It starts gradually at first, a little bit of a soft muscle tone on the torso, a slightly protruding stomach and suddenly, you look in the mirror one day, and a fat man or woman looks back at you. Permit me to say, the vast majority of weight we need to shed today was piled on because we didn't have time to look after what we were putting in our bodies.

However, there is also a genetic component to obesity too. Let me break that statement down a little. We all have that friend that always seems to be eating all the time yet does not seem to ever gain weight even without any strenuous activity in his daily routine. Conversely, you may be someone who eats relatively little, but every bit of food you seem to consume seems to go straight down to hang on your torso and belly. Why is this so? You need to understand the concept of Basal Metabolic rate, BMR to get this.

At rest, different individuals burn energy at a different rate. For instance, even if you and I are both at sleep, our body continues to utilize energy as fuel to keep vital functions such as breathing and blood circulation going on. Some people burn a relatively high amount of energy to keep these critical processes going on; others burn quite a little. The rate at which our body uses energy at rest differs from person to person, and this influences how easily we gain or lose weight.

For people with a high BMR, it means their body requires more energy (measured in calories) at rest, and they can only derive this energy from the food we eat or the excess stores that the body keeps. Therefore, they may find it harder to gain weight as their body continuously burns energy at a high rate. People with a low BMR, on the other hand, require smaller quantities of energy to keep alive. Their body can retain more fat because it doesn't have less requirement to burn energy. If two people with widely varying BMR values, eat the same quantity of food therefore and go to sleep, for instance, the one with the higher BMR will burn off more of the calories he has consumed. The individual with the low BMR would burn off smaller calories and retain the rest in the body to be stored as fat.

Now, our BMR is often determined by heredity, and there is little you can do to affect the value. However, knowing your own BMR can easily help you keep a handle on what you eat. A low BMR means you need a smaller quantity of calories to get along and a higher tendency to pile on the pounds. This does not mean people with a high BMR value should keep eating indiscriminately. With reduced physical activity, anyone will eventually turn excess food into extra weight.

Having understood BMR, let us get down to the arithmetic involved in gaining or losing weight. Food that we eat is turned into energy as measured in calories. The activities we carry out require energy to be expended, also measured in calories. Therefore, if you eat a certain amount of food calories within a period, and spend fewer calories in physical activity, you are going to have a net calorie gain, right? Where do these excess calories go? Into gaining weight is the correct answer.

On the other hand, if you expend more calories than you consume, then your body accounts for the deficit in the expenditure by burning some stored calories. That equals weight loss. Do not forget that the BMR plays a role in how much calories you get to burn. Your calorie output, therefore, is your BMR plus the extra calories you burn on physical activity.

To succinctly summarize, to lose weight, you need to expend more calories than you consume from your diet. If you consume more calories than you expend, you gain weight.

Mathematically,

Calorie input (from food) > Calorie output (BMR+ physical activity)
= weight gain

Calorie input (from food) < Calorie output (BMR+ physical activity)
= weight gain

Obesity is fast turning out to be an easily preventable yet common scourge in society today. Your BMR plays a vital role in determining the kind of body type you have. However, by choosing the right food and when to eat, you can tweak your body better to your specifications. Physical activity remains the only way to get out the calories you have consumed in food. Too little of it guarantees you will gain weight faster than if you expend more effort getting in the exercise. The right diet and physical activity is the secret to defeating obesity permanently.

CHAPTER TWO

WHY YOU SHOULDN'T BE OBESE

You started reading this book because you feel you need to know how to lose weight effectively. However, the easiest way to lose weight is not to gain that weight initially. Most people who need to lose weight would have been better served not gaining weight initially. With this in mind, here are some of the reasons why you should not watch yourself become obese before you start maintaining optimal weight for your age and body size. Being overweight or obese,

Decreases quality of life and affects health

Being obese can severely affect the quality of life you enjoy. Obese people generally find it harder to get involved in as many activities as other people. That may be the source of the obesity in the first place, but once you get overweight, it is a pretty rough road down there if you do not act immediately. Being grossly overweight is bound to affect your fitness levels and mobility. Apart from the quality of life, it can affect even the span of life. A study has found out that for every two inches you add in waistline circumference, the rate of mortality increases by 13% in women and 17% in men. If that's not a scary enough reason to find a fix immediately, I don't know what is.

Increases the chances of cardiovascular diseases

The circulatory system made up of the heart and blood vessels is undoubtedly very important in the role it plays. It pumps blood and nutrients around the body and collects waste for excretion. Being obese, however, affects its efficiency. Worldwide, more people die from cardiovascular diseases than any other health problem. Therefore, obesity as a risk factor for these diseases needs to be dealt with. How does being overweight promotes the chances one has of cardiovascular diseases?

Firstly, obese people are at increased risk of atherosclerosis, a condition where excess fats and cholesterol build up along blood vessels, narrow them and cause a less-than-optimal flow of blood through them. With time, this may lead to a shortage of blood supply to a particular area of the body and result in a stroke. Therefore, obese people are also at a higher than average risk of suffering strokes and even a complete heart attack. More so, because there is a reduction in blood vessels diameter, the heart is also forced to pump blood under more pressure than necessary. Being fat also means that there are more muscle and fat to cater for than ever before. These also need blood and the surface area that the heart supplies increase to put even more pressure on the heart. This directly translates to obese people having higher blood pressure than moderate-sized individuals. Consistently high blood pressure has dangerous implications for overall cardiovascular health.

Aids the progress of diabetes mellitus

Diabetes mellitus is perhaps the most common metabolic disease today. It is characterized by persistently high blood sugar levels. Obesity is one of the most potent risk factors for developing diabetes. In fact, it is often regarded as the sole cause of type 2 diabetes/Non-insulin dependent diabetes mellitus. Obese people often have impaired sensitivity to insulin, a hormone responsible for moving glucose from the blood into cells.

Musculoskeletal disorders

When you become overweight, more stress is placed on joints and the entire musculoskeletal system as they now have to bear the added weight. This extra weight makes obese people prone to joint pain and dislocation, especially at the knees, and ankle. Gout, while not exclusively linked to being fat, has also been found to be more common among overweight people.

Financial implications

Obesity is going to cost you much more money than being lean. In the first place, if you have grown overweight as a result of a lavish diet, then you have lost money making yourself uncomfortable. Now, to get back into shape, you are going to need to commit financial resources again. Gym subscription and equipment, weight-loss books and programs all have financial implications on you. Hell, you may even need to fork out money for a new pair of trainer shoes.

Sleep apnea

Overweight people suffer from a myriad of respiratory issues when they sleep. They often get blocked throats that wakes them up frequently (apnea) leading to uncomfortable sleeping routines. By the same measure, snoring is more rampant among the overweight especially when they get their airways blocked which happens more regularly than one would think.

Hampers social grace

More than half of everyone looking to lose weight is due to societal or peer pressure. Obesity has been derided so much in contemporary media that it is wholly understood that you may feel a little bit insecure about your body when you are obese. It is almost pointed out as evidence of ill-living, and that is the motivation for weight loss. A few extra pounds here and there, and you can soon say goodbye to tight-fitting outfits. Being overweight can even affect your self-esteem and personal confidence due to body-shaming. The importance of remaining slim and slender as a fashion preference is almost a cliché right now. It may even lead to problems of malnourishment among potential models and young adults. You can look good in whatever body shape you have, but there is no denying that your favorite pair of bikini or tailored suits look better when you do not have excess flesh hanging from your belly and upper arms.

CHAPTER THREE

CLASSES OF FOOD AND THEIR EFFECT ON METABOLISM AND BODY WEIGHT

We have discussed an overview of obesity and why you should look to lose weight. Now, let us get to the nitty-gritty of weight loss. We need food for survival. It provides us with energy for our activities and nutrients for our body to build itself and repel microbial attacks. However, not everything we eat is good for us.; there are so many varieties of food that it is imperative to understand the various classes and their effect on body weight.

Majorly, the classes of food that affect the body weight to a large extent are carbohydrates, proteins and fats. The other classes of food are usually in smaller quantities and do not necessarily affect body weight. Let us have a quick look at the digestion process. Digestion starts in the mouth with enzymes in saliva acting on the food we have eaten. This food then passes into the stomach where it is acted upon by gastric juice in an acidic environment. In the case of fats and oils, bile from the liver is also secreted to help with the process. From the stomach, it passes on to the intestine where final absorption into the bloodstream takes place. Unneeded food is then passed out as waste products.

Carbohydrates

Fifty to sixty-five percent of the average diet is made up of carbohydrates such as pasta, tubers, rice and bread. Carbohydrate gets digested to yield glucose, the body's preferred source of energy for its activities. Therefore, carbohydrate is rightly credited with providing us with fuel and rightly so. What happens though when we have an abundance of the wrong carbohydrates is a metabolic problem. Usually, the body converts carbohydrates to glucose in the bloodstream. Insulin works on this glucose to move it into the body cells where it is needed to generate energy. Excess glucose is then stored as glycogen in the liver and deposits around the torso.

Whenever we run low on glucose and require energy, the body first turns towards these glycogen stores and converts them to glucose for onward use. What then happens when an individual is guilty of overconsumption of carbohydrates even when there is no genuine need? Excess glucose at all times of course!!! This means the body will continue to deposit more and more glucose and this will eventually lead to a noticeable increase in body weight.

Again, the rate at which a meal of carbohydrate causes a surge in insulin production is also important when it comes to weight management. Highly starchy carbohydrates such as pasta and tubers cause an immediate, overarching increase in blood sugar and insulin levels when taken. In comparison, whole grains such as millet and wheat provide a more controlled rise in insulin and glucose level. Therefore, if you are looking to lose weight, it is more important that you allow whole grains to feature more as your source of glucose than starchy, highly glycemic carbs.

Fats and oils

Fats and oils contribute a great deal to cell integrity in the human body. They are also significant players in the development of the musculoskeletal system. Fat layers within the human body and around vital organs provide warmth and protection for delicate organs. In terms of weight gain and loss, they are significant players as well. Fat is stored all over the body especially in the things, abdomen and torso areas. Until you burn off some of these deposits, you will not get to lose weight. Some of the more successful diet plans are designed with this in mind; they aim to force the body to burn off fats instead of glucose as a source of energy. Aside from that, excess fat especially cholesterol can have adverse effects on the cardiovascular system. Such is the essence of fats and oil in determining total body weight that I have dedicated a subsequent chapter to it later.

Proteins

Proteins have a smaller role in weight loss compared to fats and carbohydrates. They function mainly in the repair of torn tissues and growth of new ones. That being said, if you are working on reducing weight through exercise, you need a good protein content in your diet to help you reap the benefits of your exercise and physical activity.

There are other classes of foods, but these are the three most important one as far as weight loss is concerned.

CHAPTER FOUR

THE DANGERS OF PROCESSED FOOD

They are around us everywhere, on the web, in our refrigerators and on every shelf on every shelf in every mall around us, but just how safe are processed foods for us? Processed foods refer to any food or product that has undergone industrial modification to make it appear sweeter, more attractive or tastier. They stand out as the most abundant manmade variety of goods on Planet Earth today. The processed food industry is a large one that sprang from the noble aim of preserving food for longer and making it easily accessible to as many people as possible. Sadly, the industry has grown on to become a behemoth in terms of revenue, but a real danger to our health and weight.

Why do I say so? Driven by the desire to make more profits, competitiveness sprang up among manufacturers of these foods and caution was thrown to the wind. Now, each manufacturer is focused on producing as attractive and sweet a product as possible. In trying to outdo one another, potentially harmful ingredients have crept their way into your favorite bar of chocolate and the chips you so love munching.

Here are a few broader reasons why you should shy away from processed foods if you want to maintain or lose some weight.

Excessive sugar and Salt

For the manufacturers, the idea is to get you hooked on the particular taste of their produces. What better way than to load up on sugar and watch you get addicted to their products. Sugar addiction is a real nutritional threat that can pay significant damage to your health and cause a disbalance in glucose management. It takes about five months after birth for us to acquire the ability to taste salt but sugar sensitivity seems to be born with us. That is a basis for how easily you can get addicted to sugar from the processed foods you consume. Worse, many people fail to connect sugar and the sweet taste they get so used to.

Apart from sugar, a lot of processed foods also contain high levels of salt. Salt can cause derangement of electrolyte and water balance in the body when taken above a certain level. Getting addicted to shopping for food off shelves ensures that you will cross these levels and more.

High-fat content

If the idea of weight loss is to reduce fat and carbohydrate content in food, then you will agree with me that processed foods high in fats are not the way to go. Most processed foods in high fat come with the double caveat that the fat they contain is trans-fat which is by far the more dangerous type of fats one can consume.

Poor Hunger management

If each time you get hungry, your first instinct is to whip out your packet of cornflakes and consume, then you are going to be hungrier more times than is necessary. Because they contain refined sugar, processed foods cause a massive spike in glucose level and soon enough, a sugar dump follows. This will lead to you feeling hungrier. Therefore, you will end up consuming more food than necessary to achieve satiety.

Dangerous additives and preservatives

Let us leave the effects on weight loss for some time and talk about perhaps its greatest threat in terms of mortality. Pick up any processed food and take a long look at the unending list of ingredients and artificial additives it contains. You should be worried about these additives, some of which are carcinogenic. For instance, nitrosamine, a popular preservative has been linked to a higher chance of certain cancers. If they are artificial, they do not belong within your body and should not be consumed in significant quantities.

Ready availability

Perhaps, indulging in processed food on a few occasions may not be too bad, but the idea of the manufacturers is to get you hooked and addicted. Add to that the ready availability of these processed foods, and it is easy to see how your love for them may be the sole reason you have not been deriving the intended benefits of weight loss.

CHAPTER FIVE

FATS AND OIL, TO EAT OR NOT

They are most lovely to look at; they are one of the classes of food that produce the most-savory taste when eaten yet when compared with other types of food, some fats and oils make up the most damaging, extraordinarily destructive and top harmful foods to the human body. For this reason, it is essential to know what particular types of fats and oils should be consumed and which ones should be avoided or minimized in your diet. This is not only a prerequisite for stand-out weight loss; it is a requirement for good health too.

Examples of food that contains fats and oil in large quantities are cheese, chocolates , pork , fishes with significant oil deposits (such as mackerel, trout, catfish, and salmon), all forms of oil (such as groundnut oil, olive oil, sesame oil, Canola oil, safflower oil, sunflower oil,palm kernel oil, wheat germ oil , and shea butter oil). The good news about these fats and oil class of foods is that they are a great source of energy for our activities. The bad news is that in excess quantities, some fats and oils can pose substantial health risks and lead to an increased chance of obesity.

This raises the questions; "Should fats and oils be a part of our diet at all?" and "what type of fats and oils should be included in our diet?" The answer to the latter is in the affirmative. Not only are they a good energy source, and tasty when consumed, fats are also essential in aiding cell growth. Without them, your body might find it extremely difficult to absorb nutrients, and the production of chemical messengers such as hormones will be impaired. Fats can't be avoided as they always find their way into our everyday diet from their presence in processed fast foods to their ubiquitous presence in animal products which is consumed by all except vegetarians. So, you should eat fats but only the right type.

Generally, fats and oils are classified into polyunsaturated and monounsaturated fats. Monounsaturated fat is called "good fat" as it has fewer negative effects on the cardiovascular system.

Polyunsaturated fats on the other hand which is "bad fat" can be found in pastries such as cakes, meat pies, doughnuts and macrons, and in Microwave processed foods such as French fries, popcorns and hydrogenated oils. Trans fats which are another type of "bad fat" is present in margarine and butter.

To lose weight, you do not want to overload on fats especially polyunsaturated and Trans fats. Instead, you can add some monounsaturated fats to your diet in moderate quantity. Good fat is not the culprit, bad fat is. That's what you should be getting out of your diet.

CHAPTER SIX

WHY KETOGENESIS AND INTERMITTENT FASTING ARE YOUR BEST FRIENDS

The body is an automatic system. We have evolved in such a way that our body's biochemical systems are the very best on the planet. Our body operates in such a way that it thinks of every conceivable scenario and plans ahead of it. Ketogenesis as a phenomenon illustrates this.

What exactly is ketogenesis? And why is it essential to the body and ultimately for those trying to lose weight?

Ketogenesis is a process by which the body produces fuel for its activities in the absence of sufficient glucose. When glucose levels are low such as during fasting or starvation, the body needs to find an alternative source of energy to power the brain and perform its functions. This it does by switching to stored fatty acids in the body as an alternative to glucose. By the process of ketogenesis, these fatty acids are burnt to release three types of ketone bodies; acetate, acetoacetate and beta-hydroxybutyrate.

These ketone bodies can provide the body with enough energy until the supply of glucose is reinstated. This makes ketogenesis such a useful tool for weight loss. Go hungry for a bit, allow your body to switch to ketogenesis and go into a ketogenic state, and allow yourself to burn a bit of the stored fats in your body. By alternating the periods when you are in a ketogenic state and thriving off glucose, you can get your body to burn off the excess fats you have. Ketogenesis is not a viable option to live on permanently because excess ketone bodies in circulation will lead to a state known as ketoacidosis which is less than optimal for the body system.

Fasting has become a trend for weight loss addicts, and weight loss fanatics, all over the world and for a good reason. It is not even a new idea as several faith and belief systems have advocated fasting as a body cleanser for several centuries. The whole concept of fasting as a weight loss tool is predicated upon the fact that it pushes the body into ketosis or fat-burning mode.

Now, there are many modes of fasting, but for weight loss, intermittent fasting truly stands out as being most effective. Intermittent fasting is generally very easy to do, and its results are well-documented and pronounced. With intermittent fasting, you simply miss some meals and stretch the time between the meals you take. That means you fast for a certain period and eat for the rest of the day.

Intermittent fasting is not concerned basically with what you eat but when you eat. Therefore, there are no dietary restrictions on what you can eat. Instead, the emphasis is on eating at distinct periods. This makes it a hugely-acceptable plan as you get to keep eating everything you like eating, unlike other nutritional plans

For the sake of the uninformed, it is pertinent to note that fasting is as old as human existence itself and it has been deployed by many to achieve several objectives. Early man did not every time the way we do today. Ancient man as a hunter killed what he could find and ate it. Then, he would go on a long stretch without eating anything else until he felt hungry. Then, he would begin to hunt for food again. This meant that primarily, he practiced a less-defined form of intermittent fasting but it is fasting all the same.

Fasting works on the principle of ketogenesis as I have explained earlier. When we eat, glucose is extracted from our food, and blood sugar is stored. When glucose in the bloodstream is used up, our fat stores are broken down, and we lose weight. Glycogen and ketone bodies serve as our energy source, causing a reduction in total wet weight. Also, during a fast, the levels of Human Growth Hormone, a metabolic hormone is raised causing a decrease in body weight.

There are quite a few formats that your intermittent fasting plan can follow. For instance, the 16/8 plan, the most common form of intermittent fasting advocates an eight-hour eating window and sixteen hours of fasting. Typically, the eating window extends between twelve and eight p.m during the day. Within this window, you can eat as much as you want. Once it is eight at night, you stop eating. By the next morning, you are already on an extended fast. Skipping breakfast effectively extends the fast until around noon when you eat the first meal of the day.

There are other modes too. The 4/3 model is a bit more complicated. In this format, you get to eat normally with a calorie load of between 600-700 calories for three days while the remaining four days of the week is dedicated to a committed fast. Rapid weight loss has been reported in individuals on this diet. Another equally effective form of intermittent fasting is the 24hours plan. In this plan, you eat at a particular hour and don't eat again till the same next time the next day.

Intermittent fasting is credited with allowing the body to enjoy the benefits of ketosis. Besides that, it also stimulates autophagy, the process of replacing worn-out cells and tissues. Autophagy is essential in building a healthy lifestyle. Therefore, by fasting and inducing autophagy, the body can heal faster, and you get to see the effects of exercise quicker.

Intermittent fasting has also been found to improve prognosis when it comes to cancer growth. It can also reduce the severity of tremors in Alzheimer's disease. Overall, intermittent fasting has been proven to have a positive impact on the progression of diseases such as epilepsy in children, type 2 diabetes and infertility.

Intermittent fasting can be a bit hard to adjust to, but if you genuinely desire weight loss, it is the surefire way to shed off some extra pounds. Take a look at the different plans and options available to you, and choose one.

CHAPTER SEVEN

COMMON WEIGHT LOSS DIETS

Even a cursory Google search will reveal that there are many weight loss programs and diets out there. The vast majority do not produce any consistent results though. Due to the overload of information, it becomes quite easy to get overwhelmed into subscribing to the wrong diet plan. This book will not be complete if I do not discuss a few of the more successful diet plans out there. Let us look at a few of them.

THE ZONE DIET: This diet focuses less on the calories consumed and more on the percentage balance in nutrition. A typical meal plan on the zone diet can look like this; 40 percent carbohydrates, 40 percent protein, and 30% for fats and oil, vitamins and minerals. Fruits high on sugar such as bananas and red meat are prohibited. In terms of weight loss, the diet promises a loss of two pounds the first week.

VEGETARIAN DIET: This is one of the most common diet plans in the world. Together with its sister plan, veganism, vegetarianism throws its weight behind an all-plant diet with no animal products consumed. Its case for weight loss is predicated upon the fact that most fats and oils are eliminated. Also, a proper vegetarian diet contains less amount of insulin-spike inducing sugar. There have been confirmed health benefits in existing on a vegetarian diet but its claims of weight loss are unsubstantiated yet, at best. You also have to be careful to supplement vital elements that may be missing due to the absence of animal foods such as calcium.

KETOGENIC DIET: the all-popular ketogenic diet seeks to induce ketosis as explained in this book to generate a corresponding loss in weight. It features a reduced carbohydrate intake and increased fat intake. Nuts, oil, and fish are the essential components of this diet. The ketogenic diet has recorded marked success in controlling weight.

MEDITERRANEAN DIET: This diet is also known as the bird's diet and contains a lot of whole grains, seeds, and nuts. It is of Mediterranean origin and heavily plant-based. Green, leafy vegetables (such as broccoli and spinach) and fruits feature heavily. However, a little poultry, fish and seafood are allowed. The main focus is to ensure that the diet is low fat and high in whole grains such as millet and other cereals. Only monosaturated fats from sources such as olive oil are allowed; red meat is heavily frowned upon as it contains trans fats.

ATKINS DIET: The Atkins diet as put forward by Robert Atkins in 1972, consists of very minimal carbohydrate and a higher percentage of fats and proteins. The Atkins diet sues for more satiety that can be derived from getting weaned off glucose. With the Atkins diet, weight loss is achieved by a reduction in overall calorie intake. It has been proven time after time that the Atkins diet not only promotes weight loss, it does so without raising the risks of cardiovascular diseases as most other high-fat diets seem to do.

Others forms of weight loss diets in fashion include the Slim Fast diet, The Volumetric diet, Jenny Craig diet, The Paleolithic diet and the weight watchers' diet, etc. In choosing a diet plan for weight loss, look out for comfortability, cost estimates and ease of adherence asides efficacy. Your choice of diet is important in the determination of how much pounds you get to shed.

CHAPTER EIGHT

EXERCISE AND PHYSICAL ACTIVITY, THE PILLAR OF WEIGHT LOSS

In the introduction to this book, I theorized that both diet and exercise have similar roles to play in determining if you are going to lose weight or not. Let me prove it from the mathematical formula in the first chapter.

Remember,

Calorie input (from food) > Calorie output (BMR+ physical activity) = weight gain

Calorie input (from food) < Calorie output (BMR+ physical activity) = weight gain

We need a calorie deficit to lose weight, right? Even if you reduce the calorie input you are getting from food but fail to engage in exercise that can burn off calories for you, you may not lose weight. Therefore, not only must calorie intake drop, physical activity must increase too.

Unfortunately, our daily routine or profession may mean that you get little by way of physical activity. This sedentary lifestyle as lived by people such as bankers, doctors and consumer care specialists, is a ticking time bomb for your aspirations to lose weight. Therefore, exercise exists as a way of getting as much physical activity into our daily routine as possible. By leveraging on the power of exercises, you can get to burn the required calories even with a sedentary lifestyle. For this reason, it is absolutely vital that you work regular exercise into your daily schedule. How?

The best time to exercise is in the morning before you eat. Usually, by the time we wake up, our body has fasted for six to eight hours while we sleep. That means glucose stores have been depleted and the body is burning stored fat and glycogen as fuel. Would it not be wise then to exercise, increase the demand for energy supply and accelerate the fat-burning process instantly? Exercising shortly after you wake up can help give you that fit feeling for the day's activities.

For an individual seeking to lose weight, a minimum of thirty to forty-five minutes workout is advisable each day. This does not have to be done all at once. It could be fifteen minutes in three spurts. If your mornings are too busy, I suggest you wake up just a bit earlier to accommodate exercise into your schedule.

If it is simply impossible for you to get exercise into your morning routine, then you can reschedule it for later in the day as far from lunch as possible to reap the full benefits. Now, there are one thousand and one varieties of exercise you can use to lose weight. What is most important is that you get your heart pumping faster. Below are some few tips to help you with exercise.

- Exercise does not have to be very formal. Even a long walk or light jogging for an extended period can qualify as enough exercise for a day.
- Even mowing your lawn is a form of physical activity
- Aerobic exercises help you burn more calories.
- Start simple. Get a skipping rope or hit the swimming pool to get reconditioned if you have not been getting enough exercise recently.
- Try strength and resistance training at least twice a week. Use dumbbells, weights or even your body to build your core.
- Do not exhaust yourself. Stop when you feel pain and take a little break.

Exercise is an integral part of weight loss. Diet alone cannot keep you at the optimal weight you want. Exercise helps you get to that range faster and stay there comfortably. It doesn't matter how you work it in but get more exercise and physical activity into your routine.

CHAPTER NINE

COMMON MYTHS ABOUT OBESITY DEBUNKED

A lot of myths swirl around weight loss, from the dubious to the obvious. A lot of public opinion-driven myths have come to stand the test of time yet that does not make them accurate all the same. Most of these myths have contributed a lot to areas like body-shaming and promote dangerous practices. For instance, at the beginning of this millennium, the media was agog with news about the world largest human who weighed an alarming 1300 pounds. While many were stunned by his size, others were alarmed because news spread that he got that big because he sat on a spot without moving for years. Such is the nature of unsubstantiated facts that become myths from constant repetition.

MYTH 1: OBESITY IS CAUSED BY IMMOBILITY OR LIMITED PHYSICAL ACTIVITY

Many believe that being immobile is the only reason individuals become obese neglecting other causative factors such as insufficient rest, genetically related obesity, poor hygiene and dietary conditions amongst other factors. While a lack of physical activity is bound to show negatively in weight gain, obesity is not caused entirely by limited movement and physical activity.

MYTH 2: EATING A LOT MAKES ME FAT

This is pretty similar to the first myth. The importance of food to the body can never be overemphasized, most importantly the importance of food containing the right amount of protein, carbohydrates, fats and oil, minerals and vitamins. To maintain optimal weight, it is important to eat well and eat right. Simply wolfing down everything on your plate alone though cannot turn you fat. That would depend on a lot of genetic factors too and the amount of physical activity you are getting.

MYTH 3: WEIGHT CAN BE SHED BY A BIT OF ACTIVITY

The challenge with this myth is that many have been misled into believing that no matter how careless they are with their diets, a few push-ups each morning for the next week or a run-up a hill could restore their overall body mass index. This is not too correct though as it is faster to gain calories than to lose calories. Physical activity will surely help you lose weight, but it must be of adequate quantity and sustained for long enough to have an effect.

MYTH 4: I NEED AN INSTRUCTOR TO LOSE WEIGHT VIA EXERCISE

Losing weight or shedding excess pounds can be such a painfully long and boring process which may be harder when carried out in isolation or when done alone but it is possible to lose weight without a coach, mentor or a guide. The presence of an instructor or a trained expert makes the process simpler and less confusing, but many people have lost a lot of weight with dedication as their guide and personal discipline as their only teacher.

MYTH 5: BREAST-FED CHILDREN ARE LESS LIKELY TO BE OBESE

This myth is an old tale that has gone on for too long and has settled in people consciousness as truth. There is however no scientific evidence to suggest that children who are breastfed are less likely to become obese while those who are not often end up overweight. There are certainly many noticeable and beneficial effects noticed in the children who are breastfed when compared with those who were not but obesity isn't one of them.

MYTH 6; EAT BREAKFAST ALWAYS

This is the biggest of all myths. For so long, nutrition guides screamed in our ears to eat breakfast always. We were told a thousand and one things that are wrong with not eating breakfast. Missing the first meal of the day was wrongly associated with a lot of harmful biochemical events. Luckily, recent evidence has shown that skipping breakfast actually speeds up weight loss. It prolongs the established fast that we have started deliberately or not after the last day's dinner and allows ketogenesis to go on. This leads to actual fat-burning and weight loss.

MYTH 7; EAT MANY SMALL MEALS

It was put forward as the healthiest way to eat. Eat many smaller-sized meals each day instead of larger, fewer meals. This was supposed to present the body with a steady source of energy all day and cause little fat to be stored. However, it turns out that may not be the smartest thing to do. One, eating five to six meals each day ensures that there is always some glucose just being released into the blood, leading to elevated sugar levels almost all day. More so, it matters not how many times you eat. The only thing that matters is the number of calories being consumed. Therefore, you can eat a 600-calorie in four instalments or at once. The effect on your weight will still be the same. Instead of focusing o how many times you eat, pay attention to the quantity of food you consume. That is the key to effective weight loss

CONCLUSION

Everyone is genuinely disinterested in getting fat these days, and for excellent reasons. Getting obese or overweight poses as much social awkwardness as health problems. There is virtually no benefit to be obtained in lugging around extra fat. However, getting rid of excess body weight is easier said than done. It requires commitment, dedication and the right kind of knowledge. That is precisely what I have provided in this book for you.

We get to lose weight only when our calorie output from physical activity exceeds the calorie intake from the food we consume. Therefore, you must look to reduce calorie intake at the same time as increasing physical activity. To achieve this, ketogenesis (and intermittent fasting) is an integral way of reducing the number of calories you consume each day.

Processed foods are a big NO if you want to lose weight. They contain bad calories and excess sugar and salt that can cause more than just obesity. Only healthy fats should be present in your diet; cut out the rest of the icky stuff. Just remember that what you eat is as important as how much you eat.

Exercise, on the other hand, increases energy generation and expenditure in the human body. Reducing calorie intake will work only when the calorie output is increased too. Work exercise into your morning routine to tap maximum benefits; choose physical activity always instead of comfort. Choose to walk down the stairs instead of taking the elevator. Walk that couple of blocks instead of hailing a cab. Take a stroll around your office when you have been sitting for an extended period.

Burn, burn the fat with the right diet and physical activity. They represent the pillars of weight loss. Eating the right kinds of food will help you shed off the extra pounds, but exercise will keep them off your frame permanently. Eat right, exercise well, that is the secret of weight loss!!!

GO TO THE LINK BELOW IF YOU WANT TO BE THE FIRST TO HEAR ABOUT NEW UPCOMING BOOKS AND GET DISCOUNTS ON PURCHASING YOUR VERY OWN COPY!!!

https://pages.convertkit.com/7153f10f7a/fccef3e8fc

www.ingramcontent.com/pod-product-compliance
Lightning Source LLC
Chambersburg PA
CBHW031335290526
45784CB00014B/2754